LOSE WEIGHT FAST

GINGER LEMON DETOX WATER FOR FAST WEIGHT LOSS

DAN HILD

Contents

1

The lemon ginger detox

The lemon ginger detox is a good starting point for those interested in cleansing the body a bit before heading into more potent territory where concerns detox diets. The reason why the lemonade detox diet is so popular and provides better results than other detox programs is because it uses the very astringent lemon as the main detox agent. Lemon and ginger are one of the cheapest and strongest of all alkalizing foods, and Mother Nature's anti-bacterial.

Lemon ginger detox is a good, safe bet for those who may be looking for an effective natural detox for the first time, and aren't sure what to start out with. But, as with all dietary changes, consult a doctor first. All foods have different effects on different physiologies. If you have an aversion or allergies to or from certain foods, and you may not know it, be sure to be certain before embarking on a lemon ginger detox diet, or any other diet.

2

Lemon Detox Diet

I am sure you have heard of the lemon detox diet. Even though lemon detoxing has been practiced for centuries, it is just now beginning to be recognized for its worth to human health. It has come full-circle and now everyone is flocking to the Internet to find out all about this diet. So what is the lemon detox diet? Although, they may vary they are based upon the principle of using lemon juice that is extracted from lemons to cleanse and detox the body from impurities and toxins.

In addition, many people find that detoxing with lemon juice also aids in weight-loss (hence lemon detox diet.) Some of these diets are just a lifestyle change, and others call for drastic actions. In order to choose the one that is best for you, you should conduct research and select one that is simple and yields the results that you want.

You must also be aware that all lemon detox diets are not alike, and some are not healthy- especially if they call for long-periods of fasting and promise you that you will lose 20 pounds in a week. This is not realistic, and by no means is a healthy choice for lemon detox. The viable diets that are out there, usually supply you with a step- by step guide on how to prepare for your detox, how to make the lemon juice, and explain in detail what they are for, and how they will benefit you. You want to make sure that if you do spend money on any detox products that you read the testimonials, and reviews to make sure it is not a scam.

The lemon detox diet should consist of a clear-cut plan of action, with strategic details on how to detox your body, what to expect, and with a guarantee. This is the best way to go about not losing any money, but also gaining a great insight and education on how to detox effectively with lemon juice to assure that your health is benefited fully. The right lemon detox diet can essentially boost your metabolism, enable you to lose weight safely, improve your energy and health, and allow you the convenience of affordability. If a diet you see possesses all of these characteristics- it is most likely is the right one that can get you on the path to a life without toxins and excess weight.

3

Ginger Detox And Health Benefits

Ginger is one of the best detoxifying herbs recommended in all cleansing programs including the 3 day detox diets. It's indeed brought about by nature discovered by alternative medicine experts especially in China, India and other countries practicing this way of naturally treating diseases.

According to these alternative medicine practitioners, Ginger has both the light, soothing effects for body cleanse while its nutrients strongly targets detoxification inside the body. Ironic but interesting, Ginger is also considered best detox herb so far which can be added onto different dishes, spices and even drinks nowadays in which the kitchen would never miss it in a basket.

What Are Ginger's Health Benefits?

Having been used for more than 3 centuries now, Ginger has been the favorite medicinal ingredient also considered as culinary herb. Why? Because not only by having its unique taste, unlike most spices the Ginger still retains its medicinal value while it grows under ground. In fact, it's mistaken as the "Ginger root" but it's actually Ginger's rhizome which is more likely a subterranean stem than a root.

Most of the times, people are seen using the dried ginger one but there are also powdered gingers for easy consumption helping fight digestive ailments and breaking down proteins even better. Also it's convenient because you may keep the sliced off rhizome in the refrigerator for long (around 3 weeks max) and use it for future purposes as long as it's not totally peeled.

One of the best 3 day detox benefits ginger has is the gas reduction. Most people complain about having increased gas while they enhance protein intake. But with the help of adding ginger into food, it relieves feeling bloated of gas and in turn eases nausea, motion sickness as well as feeling to vomit every morning.

Can Ginger Help Fight Away Diseases?

Yes it can. Actually it helps reduce inflammation wherein it can be used to treat diseases resulting to inflammation such as ulcerative colitis and arthritis. Additional studies show that ginger boosts anti-inflammatory through inhabitance of herpes simplex virus replication.

While detoxification enhances natural body cleansing and repairing it also allows the body to have better defenses against virus carried diseases such as fever and flu. Also, it helps stimulate blood circulation to prevent clotting which lead to chronic and deadly cases.

Thus, Ginger's healing and detoxifying properties include shogaols, volatile oils and gingerols both responsible for not only its pungent taste but also its healing processes soothing the digestive system. The volatile oils help sustain digestive enzymes which neutralizes acids and supports the whole digestion process. As a result, you can say good bye to stomach discomfort, diarrhea and even constipation.

Quick hint: One good 3 day detox diet tip for you to consider ginger's health benefits is through a ginger tea. Prepare a tea by steeping about 5 slices of ginger in hot water. Otherwise, add ginger into as many dishes as you can and combine it with lemon for best results.

4

Hints And Tips For Using The Lemon Detox Diet

Elimination

Eliminating toxins from your body is the key to a successful diet. Proper elimination will ensure that the toxins in your body will be released efficiently .Waste in your body that is not continuously removed will be reabsorbed through your system.

Try to have at least a couple of bowel movements per day. To assist with this, a mild laxative herbal tea is recommended. Drink one cup of the tea in the evening before bed and the sea salt water in the morning.

The laxative tea will help break up solid intestinal wastes, and the salt water will flush them out of the system.

The sea salt-water drink is also a great laxative and will produce a bowel movement.

Drink the sea salt water first thing in the morning. You should be attending the bathroom within half an hour. If you do not have a bowel movement after the sea salt drink, try drinking a little more or adding a little more sea salt.

Any problems which occur during the Lemon Detox Diet are usually the result of inefficient elimination.

Starting

Most people that will feel symptoms will feel them on the first two days. This is the time that toxins begin to circulate and dissolve in your system. Try to start the diet on days where you are least active so that you can have ade?uate rest if re?uired.

Li?uid intake

Countless problems may arise if insufficient li?uid is taken during the diet. You should be drinking at least 3-4 litres of li?uid (Detox drink + water) per day. This ensures that the waste material will not be too concentrated in the organs of elimination.

Headaches

Headaches are not caused by the lack of solid food intake.

Headaches are caused as toxins begin to be dissolved into your blood stream before beginning the process of elimination. It is actually a good sign that the detoxification process has begun and you are on the way to releasing harmful toxins from your body. It is actually the dissolved toxins that cause the headache and not the detox drink.

If you have had previous migraines or severe headaches in the past you may encounter these symptoms on the program. This is known as a healing crisis where parts of the body may receive more than normal symptoms due to previous ailments.

Usually these symptoms will go away after a few days with sufficient elimination. If you are not eliminating properly or not drinking enough fluids these headaches may persist. Most problems which occur during the Lemon Detox Diet are usually the result of inefficient elimination.

Try not to use any chemical painkillers. Instead try rubbing a little lavender oil on your temples, close your eyes and relax. The oil is widely used in aromatherapy to ease tension, tiredness and feelings of depression. Lavenders gentle yet powerful healing properties allow it to be used for burns and insect bites

Keep drinking plenty of water in addition the lemon detox drink. You may find it hard for the first few days but you are really doing your body a favour by eliminating toxins. If you feel that you cannot persist and the headaches are too strong you may have a panadol or the like, but do not give up as you are on your way to rejuvenating your body. You will feel much better in a few days. People who do have headaches on the program report back stating that after a few days the headaches disappear with the process of elimination.

Brushing your skin

Brushing your skin helps the elimination process by increasing blood flow and perspiration of toxins through the skin. Lightly brush over your skin with a loofah or brush.

Nausea

If you do experience nausea on the detox program is simply the effect of dissolved waste material circulating in your body before final elimination.

It is not a negative sign but in fact a positive sign that the detox is working and you are on your way to releasing stored up toxins from your body. This symptom will usually disappear after two or three days.

Drink some ginger tea or juice of ginger. Ginger is probably the best known natural remedy for nausea

Can I change the mix of the Lemon Detox Drink?

You may slightly alter the mixing ?uantities of your detox drink.

If you feel that the taste of the syrup is too sweet or strong you may add water to the recommended mixing ?uantities. For example if you want to add another half a litre of water to your recommended 2 litre batch to reduce the concentration of the syrup you may, but just remember that you will have to drink an extra half a litre (i.e. 2 extra glasses of the detox drink).Remember the most important part of the detox drink is to consume the three and a half lemons and the 140ml of syrup per day. So, it may take you 7 glasses or 10 glasses but as long as you drink this portion per day.

If you are feeling especially hungry, are being very physically active or have a high metabolism then you may wish to add more syrup to the mix. Try adding the syrup in a 3:2 or 4:2 ration to the lemon juice. Remember that the actual syrup is liquid food.

Find a mix that works for you. Some people like more syrup in the mix, some less.

Bad taste in the mouth

Rinse your mouth and brush your tongue regularly. Drinking peppermint tea will also help. Peppermint tea especially supports the cleansing process, offers relief from headaches, cleanses the palate and neutralizes any mouth or body odours that may arise

Cayenne Pepper

Cayenne pepper adds a nice zing to the drink, but more importantly it also helps dissolve built up mucus.

A recognized metaboliser, it adds heat to the system and thus stimulates circulation, helping the blood reach remote areas of the body, so important for effective cleansing and elimination.

In the case that you cannot handle the taste of the cayenne pepper you can slightly reduce the amount, or you may totally substitute the pepper for ginger.

Concluding the Program

The most common mistake is to eat too much too soon.

Since the digestive system has been resting for five to ten days, treat it carefully and considerately at the conclusion of the program. The transition from The Lemon Detox drink to regular food has to be undergone steadily.

Most people concluding the program will not feel a huge urge to eat to much. The most common mistake is to eat too much too soon. Listen to your body. It will let you know if you are eating too quickly too soon.

You should gradually return to healthy eating over three or four days.

- Day 1 after the detox: Stick with fresh squeezed fruit juices.
- Day 2 after the detox: Start the morning with juice and then try some pureed vegetable soup for lunch.
- Day 3 after the detox: Steamed or raw vegetables. Do not eat any meat, fish, eggs, bread and sweets and do not drink soft drinks during the first three days.
- Day 4 after the detox: Start eating "normally" again.

If you are coming off a shorter version of the diet you should be able to do so in one day but listen to your body. You will know if you are coming off too fast. Take your time. You will probably notice that your taste buds are much more alive after cleansing and you will really enjoy the taste and energy of juices, soups, and then vegetables.

5

Benefits of Ginger for Weight Loss

Ginger has a number of health benefits and that also qualify as weight loss benefits. The following benefits are ones that have studies to back them. There are far more benefits that have not yet been proved by science.

Ginger has been shown to be effective in lowering blood glucose levels

A number of studies have been done on the effects of ginger on blood glucose levels. Studies include studies on Diabetics as well as people suffering from insulin resistance.

One study included 88 insulin resistant, Diabetic patients. This was a double blind placebo controlled study to test the efficacy of ginger on glucose levels. The ginger group received 1 capsule of ginger three times a day. The ginger group saw a decrease of fasting glucose of 10% whilst the control group saw and increase of 21%.

It is very important to normalize blood sugar or blood glucose levels if you are trying to lose weight. High blood glucose levels can make you crave and choose carbohydrates.

That will affect your ability to lose weight or make healthy food choices.

Ginger Improves digestion and fat absorption but decreases fat storage

For those people wanting to lose weight, this is the grand slam of weight loss. We need healthy fats to produce cell walls, enzymes and hormones to keep the body healthy. Ginger not only improves digestion and fat absorption but also reduce and stops fat accumulation. So essentially ginger is a natural fat burner.

Ginger has anti-inflammatory properties

In another study ginger was found to be so powerful that it beat indomethacin as an anti-inflammatory. It is extremely important to reduce inflammation if your are trying to lose weight. Inflammation is a sign of toxins and if the liver is spending all of its time trying to detox the body, it doesn't have time to help you lose weight.

So ginger lowers blood sugar levels, improves digestion, increases fat absorption, reduces fat storage. It also helps the body get rid of inflammation. All powerful properties for anyone who wants to shed a few pounds!

6
Health benefits of Lemon for Weight Loss

Lemon is anti-inflammatory

Inflammation plays a big role in diet and your ability to lose weight. As an anti-inflammatory, lemon therefore aids weight loss by reducing and preventing inflammation within the body

Lemon Suppresses Weight Gain

In a study done on mice, lemon suppressed weight gain and fat accumulation.

The smell of lemon activate the parasympathetic

The Smell of lemons activated the parasympathetic nervous system. This means it reduces stress which will increase metabolism and organ function in general.

The parasympathetic nervous is extremely important in weight loss. The body essentially has a "ON/OFF" switch. Stress switches the body "OFF" and gets the body ready for fight or flight. In the OFF position, the body stores fats, craves carbs and switches blood flow to the arms and legs. Digestion and metabolism are switched off in fight or flight.

In the ON position, the body switches metabolism on, sends blood to the organs and gets ready for rest and digest - i.e. it switches digestion on.

You cannot lose weight if your body's switch is in the OFF position!

You can therefore rely on the power of lemon to switch on the metabolism. If you combine lemon with alternate nose breathing you can really tap into the power of the parasympathetic to rev up your metabolism. Studies on alternate nose breathing have shown that metabolic rate can be increased by up to 37%

7

Start the Day With Lemon Ginger Tea

Knowing the powerful effect lemon and ginger can have on your body, your diet, and your weight loss efforts, how to you include lemon and ginger in your diet to take advantage of these amazing effects?

On of my favorite ways to include lemon and ginger in my diet is by drinking it as a tea in winter and a refreshing drink in summer.

For the tea, I normally use green tea as a base for its weight loss and health properties, I add about a teaspoon of freshly crushed ginger to the tea and about two teaspoons of lemon juice. Make the tea to satisfy your palette. Add some Stevia or other natural sweetener if you have a sweet tooth, Ginger is a thermogenic herb. It causes the body to increase its own temperature, so in winter it helps you to stay warm and burn calories for free!

In summer, I normally add about three tablespoons of ginger and a whole sliced lemon to a jar or about two liters of water. I allow the water to stay in the fridge overnight so that the flavors and all the goodness of the ginger and lemon can steep into the water. I drink it with ice cubes made of lemon water mix. The drink is really delicious and refreshing and super healthy to boot. And of course is helps me with cravings and weight management.

8

Lemon Ginger

The bottom line is that there are a lot of herbs and spices that can help you lose weight and get healthy. Cinnamon has similar properties to Ginger in its effects on blood glucose levels. Apple cider vinegar has similar digestive properties to lemon.

Choose the ones you love eating and drinking and you will have found yourself a winning combination. The key to creating a great healthy diet is to find foods that are healthy and that you love. There are literally thousands of combinations out there and if you love eating that food or if you love that taste, then you will continue to do it - not because it takes willpower but because you want to!

That is how you create a diet that takes no willpower! And how you create one that lasts forever, By choosing the foods you love to eat and by improving your knowledge about these foods.

In group coaching we teach students to create their own perfect diet combinations so that they can experience a joyful life without having to go on a diet again

Try the Lemon Ginger 1 Week Challenge

If you enjoy the taste of lemon ginger water and the lemon ginger tea, try drinking at least three cups of two or two liters of the lemon ginger water in summer.

Try this for a week and notice the difference. Yes, there will most likely be a difference on your scale, but also notice the difference in the way you feel. You should notice an increase of energy and a decrease in fatigue. This is as a result of the anti-inflammatory and detox effects of the drink. You may find you are less "puffy" and that you are more mentally focused.

The body is an amazing machine. It is built to keep you feeling healthy and looking great. It really needs very little to make sure you love your life. Give your body a bit of attention and you will not believe the difference.

9
Reasons Why You Should Drink Ginger Lemon Tea

How to make y~~our own Fresh~~ Ginger ~~Lemon~~ Tea (which is actually an infusion, not really "tea.")

Let's see how:

1. It Boosts Your Immune System: On top of the list of benefits of ginger lemon tea is its ability to strengthen your immunity. .This is due to the presence of high levels of anti-oxidants in ginger. Lemons are an excellent source of vitamin C which can heal wounds and preserve the strength of bones and teeth. In the onset of cold and flu, the ginger lemon tea can act as an effective anti-biotic. The bioflavonoids that lemons contain help to prevent cancer cells from growing and spreading. The anti-oxidants in the lemons help in reducing inflammation and arthritis symptoms. The powerful anti-oxidants can reduce free radicals in the body. Ginger also increases blood circulation in the body that is vital for optimum health.

1. It Brings Instant Relief From Nausea and Indigestion: Vomiting and nausea usually occur as symptoms of a body disorder. Ginger lemon tea provides the best relief mechanism. Moreover, if you have a motion sickness tendency, you can drink a cup of ginger lemon tea prior to travel to prevent nausea. It can also help cure the vomiting related to chemotherapy and pregnancy, which is a relief during that period. It eases the pain and uneasiness of an upset stomach. The ginger and lemon in the tea lowers the chances of heartburn and indigestion. It causes the food to be better absorbed by the body and prevents belching and bloating after eating too much. It improves your appetite as well.

2. It Lowers The Effects Of Diabetes: New research has thrown light upon the fact that drinking ginger lemon tea on a daily basis can reduce kidney damage that occurs due to the effects of diabetes. The high levels of zinc found in ginger play a prime role in the production and secretion of insulin. It is the insulin that controls the blood sugar levels and keeps diabetes in check. Other harmful effects of diabetes like blood pressure, heart problems and so on can be countered by the anti-oxidants present in the drink.

4. It Is Your One-Stop-Drink To Perfect Skin And Great Hair: As mentioned above, ginger lemon tea is rich in anti-oxidants and vitamins which are beneficial for perfect skin, hair and health. The beverage helps in improving your digestion and guides you towards smooth and flawless skin. The antibacterial and antiseptic properties protect your skin from

infections. For strong and beautiful hair, ginger lemon tea provides you a natural aid. Vitamin A and C are recommended in plenty for those with hair issues, as they combat the production of DHT in the scalp that in turn triggers hair growth. A vitamin and anti-oxidant rich drink like ginger lemon tea will help you overcome hair problems in an absolute natural and simple way.

5. It Is The Apt Drink For Weight Loss: High blood sugar levels trigger cravings for carbohydrates and fatty foods. Ginger helps to normalize these sugar levels which otherwise can affect your ability to lose weight or eat healthy food. Ginger also improves fat absorption and prevents it from accumulating in the body. Both ginger and lemon have anti-inflammatory properties that prevent inflammations and enhance the activity of the liver that helps in shedding those extra pounds. The smell of lemons reduces stress causing an increase in metabolism and proper organ function that can help in weight loss. Lemon and ginger water will help regulate sugar levels and keep hunger pangs at bay. This prevents overeating and helps you achieve your weight loss goals in a better way. Moreover, the aroma of lemons can help reduce stress, which in turn will help you get better results from your weight loss efforts.

6. It Improves the Lymphatic System: A cup of lemon ginger tea can help keep the lymphatic system well hydrated. Lemon water is especially beneficial in stimulating the lymphatic system and this helps

eliminate toxins from the colon, lymph glands, and bladder. Ginger makes this process work even efficiently and prevents several chronic illnesses such as cancer. Regular consumption of ginger lemon tea will purify your blood and lower cholesterol as well.

7. It Alkalizes Your Body: You need to maintain an alkaline state within your body to stay healthy. When your body is in an acidic state, cancer cells are more likely to grow with ease. It is hard to achieve that state considering the toxins in the world around you – there are toxins in beauty care items, personal care items, and several household products. Lemon ginger tea will work amazingly well to create an alkaline state, which reduces chronic inflammation and prevents autoimmune diseases and illnesses, such as fibromyalgia, ankylosing spondylitis, and rheumatoid arthritis.

8. Cortisol production: Lemon ginger tea suppresses cortisol. Cortisol is a steroid hormone necessary for energy regulation and mobilization. But chronic stress can cause cortisol levels to rise too high. Adipose fat moves to the visceral area where it receives an increased blood supply that encourages tissues to produce an excess amount of cortisol. High cortisol levels may increase excess belly fat and weight gain.

10

Safety and Precautions

Side effects

Drinking lemon-ginger tea is usually safe, not causing any severe side effects. However, increased intake might cause some digestive issues due to the effect of ginger.

During pregnancy

Although it is recommended to pregnant women for relieving the symptoms of morning sickness, overconsumption must be avoided. Drinking the herbal decoction is considered safe for breastfeeding women. Make sure to consult your doctor before consuming it during these times.

11

How do we prepare ginger lemon tea?

Sliced fresh ginger root using green tea as a base, finely chop the ginger root and infuse it boiling water for twenty minutes. This helps in transferring the active ingredients into the liquid. Adding two tablespoons of lemon juice and honey or stevia into the mix helps in both sweetening the tea as well as countering the spicy effects of the ginger. It can be served either hot or cold as the revitalizing effects are the same.

Ginger lemon tea can be very refreshing to drink with its medicine like qualities. Moreover, a few recent studies suggest that it can help to stop blood clotting and lower cholesterol levels. This can prevent cardio-vascular diseases and strokes from taking place.

If you feel tensed or worn out, the drink can also be an effective stress reliever. The strong aroma, spicy and refreshing taste and calming effects provide you relief and relaxation of your body and mind.

12

Recipe: Lemon Ginger Detox Juice

Fruits are a natural partner for detoxifying our bodies. Most fruits are high in li?uid-content, which helps the body wash out toxins. Citrus fruits help flush out these toxins and jump start our digestive tracts. Lemon juice also supports the liver in its cleansing processes.

A natural anti-inflammatory food, ginger promotes detoxification by speeding the movement of food through our intestines, thanks to the compounds gingerols and shogaols.

1 serving

Ingredients

- 12 ounces water
- ½ Lemon
- ½ inch Ginger Root

Directions

1. Combine the water and the juice of the half lemon.

1. Use a zester to finely grate the ginger into the drink.

3. Stir and enjoy!

Optional: Pour over ice or add a few mint leaves.

This drink is a wonderful way to support your body's detox system first thing in the morning, but it's a natural boost any time of day.

Disclaimer

Introduction

By using this book, you accept this disclaimer in full.

No advice

The book contains information. The information is not advice, and should not be treated as such.

If you think you may be suffering from any medical condition you should seek immediate medical attention. You should never delay seeking medical advice, disregard medical advice, or discontinue medical treatment because of information in the book.

No representations or warranties

To the maximum extent permitted by applicable law and subject to section below, we exclude all representations, warranties, undertakings and guarantees relating to the book.

Without prejudice to the generality of the foregoing paragraph, we do not represent, warrant, undertake or guarantee:

- that the information in the book is correct, accurate, complete or non-misleading;

- that the use of the guidance in the book will lead to any particular outcome or result.

Limitations and exclusions of liability

The limitations and exclusions of liability set out in this section and elsewhere in this disclaimer: are subject to section 6 below; and govern all liabilities arising under the disclaimer or in relation to the book, including liabilities arising in contract, in tort (including negligence) and for breach of statutory duty.

We will not be liable to you in respect of any losses arising out of any event or events beyond our reasonable control.

We will not be liable to you in respect of any business losses, including without limitation loss of or damage to profits, income, revenue, use, production, anticipated savings, business, contracts, commercial opportunities or goodwill.

We will not be liable to you in respect of any loss or corruption of any data, database or software.

We will not be liable to you in respect of any special, indirect or consequential loss or damage.

Exceptions

Nothing in this disclaimer shall: limit or exclude our liability for death or personal injury resulting from negligence; limit or exclude our liability for fraud or fraudulent misrepresentation; limit any of our liabilities in any way that is not permitted under applicable law; or exclude any of our liabilities that may not be excluded under applicable law.

Severability

If a section of this disclaimer is determined by any court or other competent authority to be unlawful and/ or unenforceable, the other sections of this disclaimer continue in effect.

If any unlawful and/or unenforceable section would be lawful or enforceable if part of it were deleted, that part will be deemed to be deleted, and the rest of the section will continue in effect.

Law and jurisdiction

DISCLAIMER

This disclaimer will be governed by and construed in accordance with Swiss law, and any disputes relating to this disclaimer will be subject to the exclusive jurisdiction of the courts of Switzerland.

31